A CONCISE SUMMARY OF

Shred

...in 30 minutes

A 30 MINUTE HEALTH SUMMARY

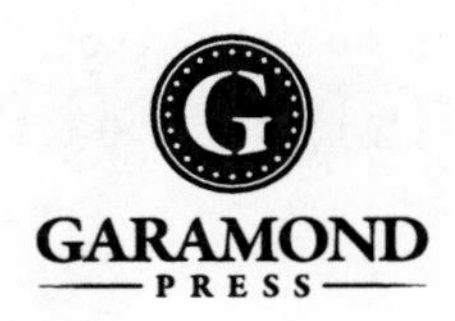

For general information on our other products and services or to obtain technical support, please contact our Customer Care Department within the U.S. at (866) 744-2665, or outside the U.S. at (510) 253-0500.

Garamond Press publishes its books in a variety of electronic and print formats. Some content that appears in print may not be available in electronic books, and vice versa.

ISBNs: 978-1-62315-090-7 Print | 978-1-62315-091-4 eBook

CONTENTS

INTRODUCTION

Overview

SHRED: The Revolutionary Diet by Ian K. Smith, MD, is a hybrid weight-loss program specially designed to help frustrated dieters break through the weight-loss plateau. SHRED combines all aspects of Dr. Smith's knowledge of dieting and weight loss into one program. He calls the plan SHRED to emphasize the way it encourages the body to shred excess fat.

The diet encompasses six weeks, which, after completion, marks the end of a SHRED cycle. Smith writes that, while many people experience dramatic results after one cycle, the diet is designed to begin again at Week 1 after those six weeks are completed—a process Smith calls *cycling*.

Each week is designated with a corresponding chapter. Within each chapter, Smith provides detailed meal plans that distribute calories over the course of the day to stave off hunger and bingeing and help stabilize hormone levels. He also outlines an exercise schedule. The SHRED program is aimed to boost dieters' willpower and motivation to make lifelong changes, and see consistent results.

About the Author

Dr. Smith's previous bestsellers include *The Fat Smash Diet, Extreme Fat Smash Diet, The 4 Day Diet, Eat,* and *Happy*. He regularly contributes to *Rachael Ray Show,* and is the host of *HealthWatch,* a nationally syndicated radio show. He served as the medical and diet expert on VH1's *Celebrity Fit Club* for six seasons and has appeared on other acclaimed television programs, including *The View, Larry King Live,* and *Anderson Cooper 360*. His articles have been published in *Time, Newsweek, Men's Health,* and the *New York Daily News*. Dr. Smith also founded two national health initiatives, the Makeover Mile and the 50 Million Pound Challenge. Since the Challenge was launched in April 2007, more than half a million people have lost a collective five million pounds. In 2010, Barack Obama appointed Smith to the President's Council on Fitness, Sports, and Nutrition.

How the Book Came About

Dr. Smith was working with a friend who had dropped almost 30 percent of her body weight but couldn't drop the last twenty pounds. Her body had grown accustomed to her new, healthier habits and she had hit a plateau. Using all he knew about strategic dieting and effective weight loss, Smith created a specialized diet plan that combined all the techniques into one program. Over the next year, he continued fine-tuning SHRED, applying feedback and criticism from users via Twitter to sharpen his approach. Published by St. Martin's Press in 2012, *SHRED: The Revolutionary Diet* became a bestseller, helping thousands of people lose weight, gain energy, and boost self-confidence.

1

THE SHRED CONCEPT

Overview

The SHRED diet combines Dr. Smith's top strategies for losing weight into one workable plan. Dieters who follow SHRED tackle frustrating plateaus, lose weight, gain confidence, and show improved health and boosted energy levels. Each of the program's six weeks targets a specific goal, from weight loss to cleansing. Together, all six weeks comprise a complete cycle. The plan carefully defines every meal and snack, and suggests specific times to eat during the day. It is designed for ease and flexibility, so that dieters (who Dr. Smith refers to as SHREDDERS) stick with the program and experience lasting results.

Chapter Summary

Shred Cycles

Six weeks make up a complete SHRED cycle—*Prime, Challenge, Transformation, Ascend, Cleanse,* and *Explode*—and each week deliberately serves a unique purpose. Prime teaches users the importance of meal spacing and proper snacking and lays the foundation for the rest of the plan. Challenge pushes comfort zones, helping users abandon bad habits. Transformation, the toughest week of the program, reveals to

SHREDDERS the benefits of their hard work: dramatic changes in weight and energy levels. Ascend reenergizes users and confirms their commitment. Cleanse detoxifies the liver, cleansing the body. Finally, Explode launches users into a life of healthful living—or if necessary, into the next cycle to continue their path to wellness. While these weeks have been created so that they can stand alone, when used together, they maximize results.

Meal Spacing

While most diets focus heavily on what foods to eat, they miss the important factor of *when* to eat. Research shows that eating meals and snacks at specific intervals keeps insulin and cortisol (two hormones released when we eat) levels more consistent as they release into the bloodstream. Doing so allows the body to lose weight more effectively and keeps it from gaining excess fat that can lead to health problems like diabetes. Properly spacing snacks and meals also helps eliminate feelings of intense hunger between meals.

Smith suggests spacing meals and snacks throughout the day according to the following schedule:

8:30 a.m.	10:00 a.m.	11:30 a.m.	1:00 p.m.	3:30 p.m.	7:00 p.m.	8:30 p.m.
Meal 1	Snack 1	Meal 2	Snack 2	Meal 3	Meal 4	Snack 3

On some days, a bonus fourth snack is added.

Diet Confusion

Muscle confusion is a principle born out of a theory that says when muscles repeatedly perform the same exercise, they eventually become so efficient that the body responds less noticeably to the exertions; in other words, the body doesn't burn as many calories, and weight loss slows or stops. However, if the routine changes on a regular basis, the muscles will continue to feel challenged, maximizing muscle gain and weight loss. The variation in workout is what causes muscle confusion. Similarly, Smith asserts that by eating a variety of foods, users can optimize *diet confusion*. Diet confusion has two benefits. First, it decreases the chance that dieters become bored with what they are eating and begin to eat off the meal plan. Second, it potentially keeps the body from becoming overly efficient at processing meals so that it continues to burn high levels of energy as it digests each meal.

The SHREDDER *Mentality*

Dr. Smith claims that dieting is 80 percent mental and 20 percent physical. The majority of dieters who fail to lose weight or give up lack the mentality required for success. Along these lines, Smith builds strategies into the program to boost willpower, discipline, and motivation. Unlike many diets that penalize users who fail to perfectly follow the program, SHRED is a forgiving plan. After completing the six-week SHRED cycle, SHREDDERS develop a mental toughness that allows them to follow through with the meal and exercise throughout the rest of their lives.

Chapter 1: Key Points

- The six distinct weeks of the SHRED plan make up a complete cycle. Many users repeatedly cycle through the program as they work toward their goals, while others may reach success after just one cycle.
- Eating meals and snacks at deliberately spaced intervals throughout the day is just as important to successful weight loss as what one eats.
- Losing weight is 80 percent mental and 20 percent physical. The SHRED program focuses not only on weight loss but also on developing strategies to increase discipline, confidence, willpower, and knowledge.

2

HOW SHRED WORKS

Overview

Dr. Smith designed SHRED so that it is easy to follow and maintain. Each week is laid out in detail so that dieters can seamlessly plan their meals. After the initial cycle, which requires close adherence, users are encouraged to customize the program to fit their individual needs and lifestyles. Food substitutions are allowed, so long as they are healthful, low-calorie foods. Once desired weight loss is achieved, users should regularly return to SHRED to review what they have learned and maintain their commitment to a healthier way of life.

Chapter Summary

Cycling

Many followers of SHRED will need to complete several cycles to reach their weight-loss and health goals. When beginning the first cycle of the program, it is important to closely follow the outlined sequence of weeks. However, on later cycles, users can customize their plan. By taking careful notes as they work through the initial cycle, they should be aware of which weeks generate optimal results and what works best for their particular needs and schedule. Most people will not complete the entire six-week cycle more than once. Dieters who have less than twenty-five pounds to lose can skip Prime (Week 1) and advance directly to Challenge (Week 2).

Exercising

Exercise is essential for maximizing weight loss. Exercise also strengthens bones, improves blood flow, increases balance and flexibility, and reduces the risk of diabetes and heart diseases. Each week of the plan calls for five days of cardio. Users should feel free to break up the recommended amount of daily exercise into two sessions, if that makes it easier for them to complete. The intensity of each exercise will determine results, so users should focus on giving as much to each workout as they possibly can. After completing the initial cycle, dieters should incorporate resistance training into their routine for twenty minutes two to three times a week.

Substitutions

While Smith conducted extensive research to formulate the meals and snacks for SHRED, he recognizes that individual food preferences, allergies, and medical conditions may prohibit dieters from eating some of the foods or drinks. To accommodate these needs, Smith encourages substitutions as long as thought and care are applied to each choice. SHRED's goal is to teach readers to make smart decisions surrounding diet by providing them with the knowledge to do so in any situation that includes food. Learning to eat foods that promote lean and healthy bodies is one of the facets that makes SHRED a lifestyle plan rather than a diet.

Maintenance

Once SHREDDERS have lost weight on the SHRED program, their goal is to keep it off. To maintain results, they must adopt the diet and exercise tools learned on the program as permanent lifestyle changes. Smith suggests closely following one SHRED week once a month—including meals and exercise—to help users stay on track. Followers should avoid choosing the same week each month. Once they have successfully kept the weight off for six months, they can reduce this practice to once every two months.

Chapter 2: Key Points

- Many SHREDDERS will require more than one cycle to reach their weight-loss and health goals. After the first cycle, SHREDDERS should use notes taken after each week of the cycle to customize their weeks moving forward.
- Exercise is critical to better health, and SHRED calls for five days of cardio per cycle. If necessary, SHREDDERS may break the required daily exercise into two sessions per day, keeping in mind that higher intensity leads to faster results.
- Food substitutions are permitted on SHRED, as long as they continue to promote success on the program.
- The true success of SHRED is keeping the weight off. To increase the chances of maintenance, readers are encouraged to choose a SHRED week and follow its menus and exercise guidelines once a month.

WEEK 1: PRIME

Overview

This week lays the groundwork for the rest of the SHRED program. Readers learn to eat meals every three to four hours, inserting snacks between meals to avoid becoming overly hungry. Dr. Smith warns against skipping meals, suggesting that if less hungry, a smaller portion is eaten at the scheduled time. Dr. Smith predicts an average weight loss of 3.5 pounds during the Prime week, but disclaims that this could be less if dieters are within twenty pounds of their target weight.

SHRED Week 1

Below is a sample schedule for recommended meal and snack times. Note that on some days there is a bonus snack.

8:30 a.m.	10:00 a.m.	11:30 a.m.	1:00 p.m.	3:30 p.m.	7:00 p.m.	8:30 p.m.
Meal 1	Snack 1	Meal 2	Snack 2	Meal 3	Meal 4	Snack 3

Guidelines:

- Record beginning weight in the morning on Day 1. This is the only weigh-in for the week.
- Eat meals every three to four hours until satiated but not until full. Do not skip meals.
- The last meal should be eaten at least 90 minutes before bedtime.
- Snacks come in between meals, and a 100-calorie snack is permitted before bedtime.
- Complete cardio exercises five of the seven days.
- This week, all shakes and smoothies shall not exceed 300 calories apiece.
- All store-bought or homemade soups are 300 calories or less this week and have no more than 480 grams of sodium per serving. Two saltines may be eaten with soup.
- One piece of fruit or one serving of vegetables must accompany all liquid meals.
- Drink a glass of water before each meal and a glass during each meal.
- One small cup of coffee per day is permitted. It should be 50 calories or less.
- A teaspoonful of ketchup, mustard, mayonnaise, or similar condiment is permitted at each meal. Spices are unlimited.

- Fresh fruit is optimal, but canned (water-based, not syrup) and frozen fruit is permitted. Canned and frozen vegetables are also acceptable.
- In addition to drinking as much water as possible, the following beverages are also permitted:
  - 1 (12-ounce) diet soda
  - Flavored waters under 60 calories
  - 1 sports drink under 60 calories
  - 1 mixed drink twice a week, or 3 light beers per week, or 3 glasses of wine per week

Meals

Dr. Smith allows two slices of 100-calorie, 100 percent whole-grain or 100 percent whole-wheat bread anytime during the day. When determining which beverages to choose, readers should opt for a different drink at each meal and mix up meals eaten during the day, keeping in mind that inducing diet confusion requires eating a wide variety of foods.

Meal 1:

- 1 piece of fruit
- Choose one of the following:
  - 1½ cups cooked oatmeal
  - 2 egg whites or 1 egg-white omelet with diced vegetables
  - 1 small bowl of sugar-free cereal with fat-free, skim, or 1 percent milk

  - 1 serving of fat-free or low-fat yogurt
  - 2 pancakes no larger than a DVD and 2 strips of bacon, 1½ tablespoons syrup and 1 teaspoon of butter
  - 1 cup cooked Cream of Wheat
  - 1 small bowl of oatmeal
  - 1 grilled cheese sandwich (use 100-calorie, 100 -percent whole-grain or 100 percent whole-wheat bread)
- 1 cup of fresh juice

Snack 1:

- 100 calories or less

Meal 2:

- Choose one of the following 300-calories-or-less options:
  - 1 fruit smoothie
  - 1 protein shake
  - 1 bowl of soup (no potato or cream)
- 1 piece of fruit or serving of vegetables
- Choose one of the following:
  - 1 (12-ounce) diet soda
  - 1 cup fresh-squeezed lemonade
  - Unlimited plain water
  - 1 cup flavored water

  - 1 cup fresh juice
  - 1 cup iced or hot tea (unsweetened)
  - 1 cup low-fat or fat-free milk, or unsweetened soy milk or almond milk

Snack 2:

- 150 calories or less

Meal 3:

- 1 chicken or turkey sandwich on 100-calorie, 100 percent whole-grain or 100 percent whole-wheat bread with lettuce, tomato, 1 slice of cheese, and up to 1 teaspoon of condiments
- 1 small green salad with up to 3 tablespoons fat-free dressing and no croutons or bacon bits
- Choose one of the following:
  - 1 (12-ounce) diet soda
  - 1 cup of fresh-squeezed lemonade
  - Unlimited plain water
  - 1 cup of flavored water
  - 1 cup fresh juice
  - 1 cup iced or hot tea (unsweetened)
  - 1 cup low-fat or fat-free milk, soy milk, or almond milk (both unsweetened)

Snack 3:

- 100 calories or less

Meal 4:

- Choose one of the following:
  - 5-ounce piece of skinless chicken (not fried)
  - 5-ounce piece of fish (not fried)
  - 5-ounce piece of skinless turkey (not fried)
- ½ cup cooked brown rice or half a baked sweet potato (1 teaspoon butter permitted)
- 1 serving of vegetables
- Choose one of the following:
  - 1 (12-ounce) diet soda
  - 1 cup fresh-squeezed lemonade
  - Unlimited plain water
  - 1 cup flavored water
  - 1 cup fresh juice
  - 1 cup iced or hot tea (unsweetened)
  - 1 cup low-fat or fat-free milk, or soy milk or almond milk (both unsweetened)

Snack 4:

- Choose one of the following:
  - 2 dates stuffed with almonds
  - 3 tomato slices topped with basil and a sprinkle of olive oil
  - 1 cup beet juice
  - 8 baby carrots with 2 tablespoons hummus
  - 1 cup unsweetened apple sauce
  - 8 dried apricot halves

Exercise:

- Time counts only when a person is moving. SHREDDERS are permitted to break sessions into two.
- Choose from the following activities:
  - Elliptical machine
  - Stationary or mobile bike
  - Swimming pool laps
  - Stair climber
  - Jogging/walking/running outside or on treadmill
  - Aerobics, including Zumba, spinning, or other high-intensity cardio
  - Rowing machine
- Feel free to increase exercise time, the more the better. Choose one program for each day of the week:

- **Day 1:** Minimum 30 minutes.
- **Day 2:** Minimum 45 minutes.
- **Day 3:** Rest day/optional extra exercise.
- **Day 4:** Minimum 40 minutes.
- **Day 5:** Minimum 40 minutes.
- **Day 6:** Rest day/optional extra exercise.
- **Day 7:** Minimum 40 minutes split into two sessions, one before 12 p.m., and the second after 2 p.m.

WEEK 2: CHALLENGE

Overview

Last week was a familiarization with the SHRED program, with mistakes surely made, meals skipped, or off-the-plan meal choices consumed. This week, the idea is to challenge readers beyond their comfort zones to stick more closely to the program. Careful attention must be made to extra calories, even seemingly minute, as they add up. This week smoothies, shakes, and soups are 250 calories or less.

SHRED Week 2

Guidelines:

- Record beginning weight in the morning on Day 1. This is the only weigh-in for the week.
- Eat meals every three to four hours until satiated but not until full. Do not skip meals.
- The last meal should be eaten at least 90 minutes before bedtime.

- Snacks come in between meals, and a 100-calorie snack is permitted before bedtime.
- Complete cardio exercises five of the seven days.
- This week all shakes and smoothies shall not exceed 250 calories.
- All store-bought or homemade soups are 250 calories or less this week and have no more than 480 grams of sodium per serving. Two saltines may be eaten with soup.
- One piece of fruit or one serving of vegetables must accompany all liquid meals.
- Drink a glass of water before each meal and a glass during each meal.
- One small cup of coffee per day is permitted. It should be 50 calories or less.
- A teaspoonful of ketchup, mustard, mayonnaise, or similar condiment is permitted at each meal. Spices are unlimited.
- Fresh fruit is optimal, but canned (water-based, not syrup) and frozen fruit is permitted. Canned and frozen vegetables are also acceptable.
- In addition to drinking as much water as possible, the following beverages are also permitted:
    - 1 (12-ounce) diet soda
    - Flavored waters under 60 calories
    - 1 sports drink under 60 calories
    - 1 mixed drink twice a week, or 3 light beers per week, or 3 glasses of wine per week

Meals

Dr. Smith allows two slices of 100-calorie, 100 percent whole-grain or 100 percent whole-wheat anytime during the day. When determining which beverages to choose, SHREDDERS should opt for a different drink at each meal. They should make an effort to mix up meals eaten during the day, keeping in mind that inducing diet confusion requires eating a wide variety of foods. Below is a sample schedule for recommended meal and snack times. Note that on some days there is a bonus snack.

8:30 a.m.	10:00 a.m.	11:30 a.m.	1:00 p.m.	3:30 p.m.	7:00 p.m.	8:30 p.m.
Meal 1	Snack 1	Meal 2	Snack 2	Meal 3	Meal 4	Snack 3

Meal 1:

- 2 pieces 100-calorie, 100 percent whole-grain or 100 percent whole-wheat bread
- 1 piece of fruit
- Choose one of the following:
    - 1½ cups cooked oatmeal
    - ½ cup cooked Cream of Wheat
    - 2 egg whites or 1 egg-white omelet with diced vegetables
    - 1 small bowl sugar-free cereal with fat-free, skim, or 1 percent milk
- ½ cup fresh juice

Snack 1:

- 100 calories or less

Meal 2:

- Choose one of the following 250-calories-or-less options:
  - 1 fruit smoothie
  - 1 protein shake
  - 1 vegetable shake using any vegetables
  - 1 bowl of soup (no potato or cream)
- 1 piece of fruit or 1 serving of vegetables.
- Choose one of the following:
  - 1 (12-ounce) diet soda
  - 1 cup fresh-squeezed lemonade
  - Unlimited plain water
  - 1 cup flavored water
  - 1 cup fresh juice
  - 1 cup iced or hot tea (unsweetened)
  - 1 cup low-fat or fat-free milk, or soy milk or almond milk (both unsweetened)

Snack 2:

- 150 calories or less

Meal 3:

- Choose from Meal A *or* Meal B:

Meal A:

- ½ cup cooked brown rice or half a baked sweet potato (one teaspoon butter permitted)
- 1 serving of vegetables
- Choose one of the following:
    - 5-ounce piece of skinless chicken (not fried)
    - 5-ounce piece of fish (not fried)
    - 5-ounce piece of skinless turkey (not fried)

Meal B:

- 1 serving (4 x 2 x 1 –inch piece) of lasagna
- 1 serving of vegetables
- Choose one of the following:
    - 1 (12-ounce) diet soda
    - 1 cup fresh-squeezed lemonade
    - Unlimited plain water
    - 1 cup flavored water
    - 1 cup fresh juice
    - 1 cup iced or hot tea (unsweetened)

- 1 cup low-fat or fat-free milk, or soy milk or almond milk (both unsweetened).

Snack 3:

- 100 calories or less

Meal 4:

- Choose one of the following 250-calories-or-less options:
    - 1 fruit smoothie
    - 1 protein shake
    - 1 bowl of soup (no potato or cream)
- 1 piece of fruit or 1 serving of vegetables
- Choose one of the following:
    - 1 (12-ounce) diet soda
    - 1 cup fresh-squeezed lemonade
    - Unlimited plain water
    - 1 cup flavored water
    - 1 cup fresh juice
    - 1 cup iced or hot tea (unsweetened)
    - 1 cup low-fat or fat-free milk, or soy milk or almond milk (both unsweetened)

Snack 4:

- Choose one of the following:
    - 20 almonds
    - 2 rice cakes with 1 teaspoon peanut butter
    - 8 dried apricot halves
    - 2 tablespoons sunflower seeds
    - 4 whole-grain or whole-wheat Melba toast slices

Exercise:

- Time counts only when a person is moving. SHREDDERS are permitted to break sessions into two.
- Choose from the following activities:
    - Jogging/walking/running outside or on treadmill
    - Stationary or mobile bike
    - Swimming pool laps
    - Stair climber
    - Elliptical machine
    - Treadmill walk/run intervals
    - Aerobics, including Zumba, spinning, or other high-intensity cardio
    - Rowing machine

- Feel free to increase exercise time, the more the better. Choose one program for each day of the week:
    - **Day 1**: Minimum 40 minutes.
    - **Day 2**: Minimum 45 minutes.
    - **Day 3**: Minimum 30 minutes.
    - **Day 4**: Rest day/optional extra exercise.
    - **Day 5**: Minimum 40 minutes.
    - **Day 6**: Minimum 30 minutes.
    - **Day 7**: Rest day/optional extra exercise.

5

WEEK 3: TRANSFORMATION

Overview

This week is the most challenging of the program. As the body adjusts to the diet and exercise habits, weight loss may slow or even plateau; therefore, the Transformation week is designed to help dieters push past this plateau. Exercise is critical this week, so Dr. Smith asks readers to give extra effort to each workout. Additionally, this week the calorie count for smoothies, shakes, and soups decreases from 250 to 200 calories. If a serving size exceeds this limit, SHREDDERS should not eat the entire portion.

SHRED Week 3

Guidelines:

- Record beginning weight in the morning on Day 1. This is the only weigh-in for the week.
- Eat meals every three to four hours until satiated but not until full. Do not skip meals.
- The last meal should be eaten at least 90 minutes before bedtime.

- Snacks come in between meals, and a 100-calorie snack is permitted before bedtime.
- Complete cardio exercises five of the seven days.
- This week all shakes and smoothies shall not exceed 200 calories.
- All store-bought or homemade soups are 200 calories or less this week and have no more than 480 grams of sodium per serving. Two saltines may be eaten with soup.
- One piece of fruit or one serving of vegetables must accompany all liquid meals.
- Drink a glass of water before each meal and a glass during each meal.
- One small cup of coffee per day is permitted. It should be 50 calories or less.
- A teaspoonful of ketchup, mustard, mayonnaise, or similar condiment is permitted at each meal. Spices are unlimited.
- Fresh fruit is optimal, but canned (water-based, not syrup) and frozen fruit is permitted. Canned and frozen vegetables are also acceptable.
- In addition to drinking as much water as possible, the following beverages are also permitted:
    - 1 (12-ounce) diet soda
    - Flavored waters under 60 calories
    - 1 sports drink under 60 calories
    - 1 mixed drink twice a week, or 3 light beers per week, or 3 glasses of wine per week

Meals

SHREDDERS should opt for different beverages with meals throughout the day and make an effort to mix up the meals eaten during the day. To induce diet confusion, a wide variety of foods should be consumed. Below is a sample schedule for recommended meal and snack times. Note that on some days there is a bonus snack.

8:30 a.m.	10:00 a.m.	11:30 a.m.	1:00 p.m.	3:30 p.m.	7:00 p.m.	8:30 p.m.
Meal 1	Snack 1	Meal 2	Snack 2	Meal 3	Meal 4	Snack 3

Meal 1:

- 1 (8-ounce) cup lemon water (½ teaspoon sugar optional)
- 1 piece of fruit or ½ cup of berries
- Choose one of the following:
    - 1½ cups cooked oatmeal
    - 2 egg whites or 1 egg-white omelet with diced vegetables
    - 1 small bowl sugar-free cereal with fat-free, skim, or 1 percent milk
    - 1 grilled cheese on 100 percent whole-grain or 100 percent whole-wheat bread
    - 1 small bowl of Cream of Wheat or grits
- ½ cup fresh-squeezed grapefruit, apple, or orange juice

Snack 1:

- 100 calories or less

Meal 2:

- Choose one of the following 200-calories-or-less options:
    - 1 fruit smoothie
    - 1 protein shake
- 1 piece of fruit or 1 serving of leafy greens or 1 serving of vegetables
- Choose one of the following:
    - 1 (12-ounce) diet soda
    - 1 cup fresh-squeezed lemonade
    - Unlimited plain water
    - 1 cup flavored water
    - 1 cup fresh juice
    - 1 cup iced or hot tea (unsweetened)
    - 1 cup low-fat or fat-free milk, or soy milk or almond milk (both unsweetened)

Snack 2:

- 150 calories or less

Meal 3:

- Choose one of the following 200-calories-or-less options:
    - 1 milk shake
    - 1 fruit smoothie
    - 1 protein shake
    - 1 vegetable shake using any vegetables
    - 1 bowl of soup (no potato or cream)
- Choose one of the following:
    - 1 (12-ounce) diet soda
    - 1 cup fresh-squeezed lemonade
    - Unlimited plain water
    - 1 cup flavored water
    - 1 cup fresh juice
    - 1 cup iced or hot tea (unsweetened)
    - 1 cup low-fat or fat-free milk, or soy milk or almond milk (both unsweetened)

Snack 3:

- 100 calories or less

Meal 4:

- 1 cup beans (not baked)
- Choose one of the following 200-calories-or-less options:
  - 1 fruit smoothie
  - 1 protein shake
  - 1 vegetable shake
- Choose one of the following:
  - 1 (12-ounce) diet soda
  - 1 cup fresh-squeezed lemonade
  - Unlimited plain water
  - 1 cup flavored water
  - 1 cup fresh juice
  - 1 cup iced or hot tea (unsweetened)
  - 1 cup low-fat or fat-free milk, or soy milk or almond milk (both unsweetened)

Snack 4:

- Choose one of the following:
  - 20 almonds
  - 2 rice cakes with 1 teaspoon peanut butter
  - Small fruit cup (no syrup)

  - 8 dried apricot halves
  - 2 tablespoons sunflower seeds
  - 4 whole-grain or whole-wheat Melba toast slices

Exercise:

- Time counts only when a person is moving. SHREDDERS are permitted to break sessions into two.
- Choose from the following activities:
  - Jogging/walking/running outside or on treadmill
  - Stationary or mobile bike
  - Swimming pool laps
  - Stair climber
  - Elliptical machine
  - Treadmill walk/run intervals
  - Aerobics, including Zumba, spinning, or other high-intensity cardio
  - Rowing machine
- Feel free to increase exercise time, the more the better. Choose one program for each day of the week:
  - **Day 1:** Minimum 40 minutes.
  - **Day 2:** Minimum 45 minutes.
  - **Day 3:** Minimum 30 minutes.

- **Day 4**: Rest day/optional extra exercise.
- **Day 5**: Minimum 40 minutes.
- **Day 6**: Rest day/optional extra exercises.
- **Day 7**: Minimum 40 minutes split into two sessions, one before 12 p.m., and the second after 2 p.m.

6

WEEK 4: ASCEND

Overview

Smith likens the first three weeks of SHRED to sliding into a dark pit. On this fourth week, dieters ascend into the light. Using everything they have learned in the first three weeks, they continue to exercise strength and willpower to work toward their weight-loss and health goals. Smoothies, shakes, and soups remain at 200 calories or less this week; readers should continue to be mindful of serving size so that they do not inadvertently consume extra calories.

SHRED Week 4

Guidelines:

- Record beginning weight in the morning on Day 1. This is the only weigh-in for the week.
- Eat meals every three to four hours until satiated but not until full. Do not skip meals.
- The last meal should be eaten at least 90 minutes before bedtime.

- Snacks come in between meals, and a 100-calorie snack is permitted before bedtime.
- Complete cardio exercises five of the seven days.
- This week all shakes and smoothies shall not exceed 200 calories.
- All store-bought or homemade soups are 200 calories or less this week and have no more than 480 grams of sodium per serving. Two saltines may be eaten with soup.
- One piece of fruit or one serving of vegetables must accompany all liquid meals.
- Drink a glass of water before each meal and a glass during each meal.
- One small cup of coffee per day is permitted. It should be 50 calories or less.
- A teaspoonful of ketchup, mustard, mayonnaise, or similar condiment is permitted at each meal. Spices are unlimited.
- Fresh fruit is optimal, but canned (water-based, not syrup) and frozen fruit is permitted. Canned and frozen vegetables are also acceptable.
- In addition to drinking as much water as possible, the following beverages are also permitted:
    - 1 (12-ounce) diet soda
    - Flavored waters under 60 calories
    - 1 sports drink under 60 calories
    - 1 mixed drink twice a week, or 3 light beers per week, or 3 glasses of wine per week

Meals

SHREDDERS should opt for different beverages with meals throughout the day and make an effort to mix up the meals eaten during the day. To induce diet confusion, a wide variety of foods should be consumed. Below is a sample schedule for recommended meal and snack times. Note that on some days there is a bonus snack.

8:30 a.m.	10:00 a.m.	11:30 a.m.	1:00 p.m.	3:30 p.m.	7:00 p.m.	8:30 p.m.
Meal 1	Snack 1	Meal 2	Snack 2	Meal 3	Meal 4	Snack 3

Meal 1:

- 1 (8-ounce) cup lemon water (½ teaspoon sugar optional)
- 1 piece of fruit or ½ cup berries
- Choose one of the following:
    - 1½ cups cooked oatmeal
    - 2 egg whites or 1 egg-white omelet with diced vegetables
    - 1 small bowl sugar-free cereal with fat-free, skim, or 1 percent milk
    - 1 grilled cheese on 100 percent whole-grain or 100 percent whole-wheat bread
- ½ cup fresh juice

Snack 1:

- 100 calories or less

Meal 2:

- Choose one of the following 200-calories-or-less options:
  - 3 servings of vegetables
  - 1 large green salad with no more than 4 tablespoons fat-free dressing (no croutons or bacon bits)
  - 1 fruit smoothie
  - 1 protein shake
  - 1 bowl of soup (no potato or cream)
- Choose one of the following:
  - 1 (12-ounce) diet soda
  - 1 cup fresh-squeezed lemonade
  - Unlimited plain water
  - 1 cup flavored water
  - 1 cup fresh juice
  - 1 cup unsweetened tea
  - 1 cup low-fat or fat-free milk, or soy milk or almond milk (both unsweetened)

Snack 2:

- 150 calories or less

Meal 3:

- Choose one of the following:
  - 5-ounce piece of lean beef (not fried)
  - 5-ounce piece of skinless chicken (not fried)
  - 5-ounce piece of fish (not fried)
  - 5-ounce piece of skinless turkey (not fried)
  - 1 cup of spaghetti and meatballs
- 1 serving of vegetables
- ½ baked sweet potato (1 teaspoon butter permitted) or ½ cup rice (brown is preferable)
- Choose one of the following:
  - 1 (12-ounce) diet soda
  - 1 cup fresh-squeezed lemonade
  - Unlimited plain water
  - 1 cup flavored water
  - 1 cup fresh juice
  - 1 cup iced or hot tea (unsweetened)
  - 1 cup low-fat or fat-free milk, or soy milk or almond milk (both unsweetened)

Snack 3:

- 100 calories or less

Meal 4:

- Choose one of the following 200-calorie-or-less options:
    - 1 fruit smoothie
    - 1 protein shake
    - 1 bowl of soup (no potato or cream)
- Choose one of the following:
    - 1 (12-ounce) diet soda
    - 1 cup fresh-squeezed lemonade
    - Unlimited plain water
    - 1 cup flavored water
    - 1 cup fresh juice
    - 1 cup iced or hot tea (unsweetened)
    - 1 cup low-fat or fat-free milk, or soy milk or almond milk (both unsweetened)

Snack 4:

- Choose one of the following:
    - 20 almonds
    - 1 large cucumber with 2 tablespoons fat-free dressing
    - Small fruit cup
    - 8 dried apricot halves

- 1 scoop of ice cream (½ cup or less)
- 4 whole-grain or whole-wheat Melba toast slices

Exercise:

- Time counts only when a person is moving. SHREDDERS should feel free to break sessions into two.
- Choose from the following activities:
    - Jogging/walking/running outside or on treadmill
    - Stationary or mobile bike
    - Swimming pool laps
    - Stair climber
    - Elliptical machine
    - Treadmill walk/run intervals
    - Aerobics, including Zumba, spinning, or other high-intensity cardio
    - Rowing machine
- Feel free to increase exercise time, the more the better. Choose one program for each day of the week:
    - **Day 1:** Minimum 30 minutes. Choose a combination of two of the exercises listed for 15 minutes each.
    - **Day 2:** Minimum 45 minutes. Choose a combination of three of the exercises listed for 15 minutes each.
    - **Day 3:** Rest day/optional extra exercise.

- **Day 4**: Minimum 30 minutes. Choose a combination of two of the exercises listed for 15 minutes each.
- **Day 5**: Minimum 45 minutes. Choose a combination of three of the exercises listed for 15 minutes each.
- **Day 6**: Rest day/optional extra exercise.
- **Day 7**: Minimum 45 minutes split into two sessions, one before 12 p.m., and the second after 2 p.m. Choose a combination of three of the exercises listed for 15 minutes each.

WEEK 5: CLEANSE

Overview

This week focuses on cleansing the body by eating foods that naturally detoxify the liver. This is known as an *eating detox*, during which SHREDDERS feel their gastrointestinal tract working more smoothly, experience a boost in energy, and notice a healthier glow to their skin. Dr. Smith asks readers to avoid substitutions, as every meal and beverage outlined is essential to the cleanser's success. Readers are given specific vegetable lists to choose from. Cleansers also add one cup of hibiscus tea, one glass of lemon water for breakfast, and one glass of cranberry juice each day. Additionally, alcohol is off-limits this week. The calorie guidelines for soups, shakes, and smoothies vary. Snack choices this week are also more defined than they were in previous weeks.

SHRED Week 5

Guidelines:

- Record beginning weight in the morning on Day 1. This is the only weigh-in for the week.
- Eat meals every three to four hours until satiated but not until full. Do not skip meals.

- The last meal should be eaten at least 90 minutes before bedtime.
- Snacks come in between meals, and a 100-calorie snack is permitted before bedtime.
- Complete cardio exercises five of the seven days.
- This week all shakes and smoothies have different calorie counts.
- The calorie counts on soups also vary. They should continue to have no more than 480 grams of sodium per serving. These may be eaten with two saltines.
- One piece of fruit or one serving of vegetables must accompany all liquid meals.
- Drink a glass of water before each meal and a glass during each meal.
- One small cup of coffee per day is permitted. It should be 50 calories or less.
- A teaspoonful of ketchup, mustard, mayonnaise, or similar condiment is permitted at each meal. Spices are unlimited.
- Fresh fruit is optimal, but canned (water-based, not syrup) and frozen fruit is permitted. Canned and frozen vegetables are also acceptable.
- No alcohol may be consumed this week.
- In addition to drinking as much water as possible, the following beverages are also permitted:
  - 1 (12-ounce) diet soda

- Flavored waters under 60 calories
- 1 sports drink under 60 calories

Meals

SHREDDERS should opt for different beverages with meals throughout the day and make an effort to mix up the meals eaten during the day. To induce diet confusion, a wide variety of foods should be consumed. Below is a sample schedule for recommended meal and snack times. Note that on some days there is a bonus snack.

8:30 a.m.	10:00 a.m.	11:30 a.m.	1:00 p.m.	3:30 p.m.	7:00 p.m.	8:30 p.m.
Meal 1	Snack 1	Meal 2	Snack 2	Meal 3	Meal 4	Snack 3

Meal 1:

- 1 (8-ounce) cup hot or cold lemon water with 2 tablespoons ground flaxseeds or flaxseed oil
- 1 piece of fruit or ½ cup berries
- Choose one of the following:
  - 1½ cups cooked oatmeal
  - 2 egg whites or 1 egg-white omelet with diced vegetables
  - 1 small bowl sugar-free cereal with fat-free, skim, or 1 percent milk
- ½ cup fresh juice

Snack 1:

- Choose one of the following:
  - 14 raw almonds
  - ½ cucumber with 2 tablespoons hummus
  - 8 baby carrots with 2 tablespoons hummus
  - 1 celery stalk with 2 tablespoons hummus

Meal 2:

- 1 cup 100 percent fresh cranberry juice (dilute to reduce bitterness, if desired)
- Choose one of the following:
  - 3 servings of vegetables (1 serving must be leafy greens)
  - 1 large green salad with no more than 4 tablespoons fat-free dressing (no croutons or bacon bits)
  - 1 cup brown rice or ½ cup beans with quinoa
- Choose one of the following:
  - 1 cup fresh-squeezed lemonade
  - Unlimited plain water
  - 1 cup flavored water
  - 1 cup fresh juice
  - 1 cup iced or hot tea (unsweetened)

Snack 2:

- Choose one of the following:
  - 2 dates stuffed with almonds
  - 10 cherries mixed with a handful of cashews, almonds, or walnuts
  - Small beet salad
  - ½ cup raisins mixed with raw walnuts and a pinch of sea salt
  - 1 cup unsweetened apple sauce

Meal 3:

- Choose one of the following 250-calories-or-less options:
  - 1 milk shake
  - 1 fruit smoothie
  - 1 protein shake
  - 1 vegetable shake with any vegetables
  - 1 bowl of soup (no potato or cream)
- Choose one of the following:
  - 1 (12-ounce) diet soda
  - 1 cup fresh-squeezed lemonade
  - Unlimited plain water
  - 1 cup flavored water

- 1 cup fresh juice
- 1 cup iced or hot tea (unsweetened)

Snack 3:

- Choose one of the following:
    - ½ cup raw nuts with sunflower or pumpkin seeds and dried fruit
    - 3 tomato slices topped with basil and olive oil sprinkle
    - 2 celery sticks with 1 tablespoon raw nut butter and 1 tablespoon organic raisins
    - 1 piece of medium-size fruit

Meal 4:

- 1 cup hibiscus tea
- Choose one of the following:
    - 5-ounce piece of lean beef (not fried)
    - 5-ounce piece of skinless chicken (not fried)
    - 5-ounce piece of fish (not fried)
    - 5-ounce piece of skinless turkey (not fried)
    - 1 cup spaghetti and meatballs
- 1 serving of vegetables
- ½ baked sweet potato (1 teaspoon butter permitted) or ½ cup rice (brown is preferable)

- Choose one of the following:
    - 1 cup fresh-squeezed lemonade
    - Unlimited plain water
    - 1 cup flavored water
    - 1 cup fresh juice
    - 1 cup unsweetened tea
    - 1 cup low-fat or fat-free milk, or soy milk or almond milk (both unsweetened)

Snack 4:

- Choose one of the following:
    - 20 almonds
    - 1 large cucumber with 2 tablespoons fat-free dressing
    - Small fruit cup
    - 8 dried apricot halves
    - Small beet salad
    - 4 whole-grain or whole-wheat Melba toast slices

Exercise:

- Time counts only when people are moving. SHREDDERS should feel free to break sessions into two.

- Choose one of the following activities:
  - Jogging/walking/running outside or on treadmill
  - Elliptical machine
  - Stationary or mobile bike
  - Swimming pool laps
  - Stair climber
  - Treadmill walk/run intervals
  - Aerobics, including Zumba, spinning, or other high-intensity cardio
  - Rowing machine
- Feel free to increase your exercise time, the more the better. Choose one program for each day of the week:
  - **Day 1**: Minimum 30 minutes. Choose a combination of two of the exercises listed for 15 minutes each.
  - **Day 2:** Minimum 45 minutes. Choose a combination of three of the exercises listed for 15 minutes each.
  - **Day 3:** Rest day/optional extra exercise.
  - **Day 4:** Minimum 45 minutes. Choose a combination of three of the exercises listed for 15 minutes each.
  - **Day 5:** Minimum 45 minutes. Choose a combination of three of the exercises listed for 15 minutes each.
  - **Day 6:** Rest day/optional extra exercise.

- **Day 7:** Minimum 45 minutes split into two sessions, one before 12 p.m., and the second after 2 p.m. Choose a combination of three of the exercises listed for 15 minutes each.

WEEK 6: EXPLODE

Overview

At this point in the SHRED program, SHREDDERS report a considerable amount of weight lost, and energy and confidence gained. Dr. Smith recommends reflecting on the past five weeks and the accompanying emotions, successes, and failures experienced. Some people will be finished with SHRED after this final week. Others will begin a new cycle. Calorie counts for smoothies, shakes, and soups vary this week. Additionally, during Explode, Dr. Smith allows *three* slices of 100-calorie, 100 percent whole-grain or 100 percent whole-wheat anytime during the day. There are also two days of exercise this week that *must* be split into two sessions, even if a person has not done so throughout the program. Readers should continue with the goal of diet confusion, making sure not to eat the same meal, shake, or smoothie more than once a day. While alcohol is permitted, dieters should be mindful of consumption.

SHRED Week 6

Guidelines:

- ➢ Record beginning weight in the morning on Day 1. This is the only weigh-in for the week.

- Eat meals every three to four hours until satiated but not until full. Do not skip meals.
- The last meal should be eaten at least 90 minutes before bedtime.
- Snacks come in between meals, and a 100-calorie snack is permitted before bedtime.
- Complete cardio exercises five of the seven days.
- This week all shakes and smoothies have different calorie counts.
- The calorie counts on soups also vary. They should continue to have no more than 480 grams of sodium per serving. These may be eaten with two saltines.
- One piece of fruit or one serving of vegetables must accompany all liquid meals.
- Drink a glass of water before each meal and a glass during each meal.
- One small cup of coffee per day is permitted. It should be 50 calories or less.
- A teaspoonful of ketchup, mustard, mayonnaise, or similar condiment is permitted at each meal. Spices are unlimited.
- Fresh fruit is optimal, but canned (water-based, not syrup) and frozen fruit is permitted. Canned and frozen vegetables are also acceptable.
- In addition to drinking as much water as possible, the following beverages are also permitted:

- 1 (12-ounce) diet soda
- Flavored waters under 60 calories
- 1 sports drink under 60 calories
- 1 mixed drink twice a week, or 3 light beers per week, or 3 glasses of wine per week

Meals

This week, Dr. Smith allows *three* slices of 100-calorie, 100 percent whole-grain or 100 percent whole-wheat anytime during the day. When determining which beverages and foods to consume throughout the day, SHREDDERS should mix up meals, keeping in mind that inducing diet confusion requires eating a wide variety of foods.

Below is a sample schedule for recommended meal and snack times. Note that on some days there is a bonus snack.

8:30 a.m.	10:00 a.m.	11:30 a.m.	1:00 p.m.	3:30 p.m.	7:00 p.m.	8:30 p.m.
Meal 1	Snack 1	Meal 2	Snack 2	Meal 3	Meal 4	Snack 3

Meal 1:

- Choose one of the following 200-calories-or-less options:
  - 1 fruit smoothie
  - 1 protein shake
  - 1 vegetable shake with any vegetables
  - 1 (6-ounce) fat-free or low-fat yogurt
- 1 piece of fruit

Snack 1:

- 150 calories or less

Meal 2:

- 1 chicken or turkey sandwich on 100 percent whole-grain or 100 percent whole-wheat bread with lettuce and tomato, 1 slice of cheese, and up to 1 teaspoon condiments
- 1 small garden salad with up to 3 tablespoons fat-free dressing and no croutons or bacon bits
- Choose one of the following:
  - 1 (12-ounce) diet soda
  - 1 cup fresh-squeezed lemonade
  - Unlimited plain water
  - 1 cup flavored water
  - 1 cup fresh juice
  - 1 cup iced or hot tea (unsweetened)
  - 1 cup low-fat or fat-free milk, or soy milk or almond milk (both unsweetened)

Snack 2:

- 100 calories or less

Meal 3:

- Choose one of the following 200-calories-or-less options:
    - 1 milk shake
    - 1 fruit smoothie
    - 1 protein shake
    - 1 vegetable shake with any vegetables
    - 1 bowl of soup (no potato or cream)
- Choose one of the following:
    - 1 (12-ounce) diet soda
    - 1 cup fresh-squeezed lemonade
    - Unlimited plain water
    - 1 cup flavored water
    - 1 cup fresh juice
    - 1 cup iced or hot tea (unsweetened)

Snack 3:

- 100 calories or less

Meal 4:

- Choose one of the following:
    - 1 small bowl of pasta with marinara sauce
    - 2 small-to-medium slices of pizza (1/16 of a pie)

    - 1 bowl of soup (no potato or cream)
    - 5-ounce piece of skinless turkey (not fried)
    - 5-ounce piece of skinless chicken (not fried)
    - 5-ounce piece of fish (not fried)
- Choose one of the following:
    - 12 thinly cut French fries or 6 steak fries
    - 1 serving of vegetables
    - Small garden salad
- Choose one of the following:
    - 1 (12-ounce) diet soda
    - 1 cup fresh-squeezed lemonade
    - Unlimited plain water
    - 1 cup flavored water
    - 1 cup fresh juice
    - 1 cup iced or hot tea (unsweetened)

Snack 4:

- Choose one of the following:
    - ½ cup raw nuts with sunflower or pumpkin seeds and dried fruit
    - 10 cherries mixed with a handful of cashews, almonds, or walnuts

- 8 dried apricot halves
- 4 whole-wheat or whole-grain Melba toast slices
- 8 baby carrots with 2 tablespoons hummus

Exercise:

- Time counts only when a person is moving. SHREDDERS should feel free to break sessions into two. However, even if one hasn't chosen to do so up to this point on SHRED, there are two days this week that Dr. Smith says *must* be split.
- Choose from the following activities:
  - Jogging/walking/running outside or on treadmill
  - Elliptical machine
  - Stationary or mobile bike
  - Swimming pool laps
  - Stair climber
  - Aerobics, including Zumba, spinning, or other high-intensity cardio
  - Rowing machine
- Feel free to increase your exercise time, the more the better. Choose one program for each day of the week:
  - **Day 1:** Minimum 30 minutes. Choose a combination of two of the exercises listed for 15 minutes each.

- **Day 2:** Minimum 45 minutes split into two sessions, one before 12 p.m., and the second after 2 p.m. Choose a combination of three of the exercises listed for 15 minutes each.
- **Day 3:** Rest day/Optional extra exercise.
- **Day 4:** Minimum 45 minutes. Choose a combination of three of the exercises listed for 15 minutes each.
- **Day 5:** Minimum 30 minutes. Choose a combination of two of the exercises listed for 15 minutes each.
- **Day 6:** Rest day/Optional extra exercises.
- **Day 7:** Minimum 30 minutes split into two sessions, one before 12 p.m., and the second after 2 p.m. Choose a combination of two of the exercises listed above for 15 minutes each.

9

SHRED SNACKS

Overview

Eating snacks throughout the day is an important part of any weight-loss program. By eating small amounts (100 to 150 calories) between meals, it is possible to stave off intense hunger that can lead to overeating or unhealthy food choices. Snacks also help to distribute calories throughout the day so that the body's hormone levels remain consistent. It's important to not overindulge with snacks, because doing so can quickly add excess calories to the daily count. Dr. Smith explains that snacks should be a bridge between meals, not a meal themselves. Choices like potato chips and cookies should be avoided; choose healthier options that provide valuable vitamins and nutrients. The SHRED program recommends consuming three to four snacks every day. In this chapter, Smith provides a list of low-calorie snack options.

Chapter Summary

The following is a list of 150-calorie snacks recommended by Dr. Smith:

- 1 cup whole strawberries dipped in 1 tablespoon melted semisweet chocolate chips
- 3 Wheat Thins with 2 tablespoons spreadable light cheese

- ¼ cup low-fat cottage cheese with ¼ cup fresh pineapple
- 7 olives stuffed with 1 tablespoon blue cheese
- 5 pieces of brown rice vegetable sushi rolls
- Nature Valley Oats 'n Honey crunchy granola bar
- ½ cup fruit sorbet topped with ½ cup blueberries
- Whole-wheat English muffin topped with 1 tablespoon tomato sauce, 1 tablespoon low-fat cheese, and 1 tablespoon parmesan cheese, and then broiled
- 15 baked Tostitos Scoops with 2 tablespoons bean dip
- ½ medium avocado sprinkled with sea salt
- 2 squares of graham crackers and 8 ounces of skim milk
- 1½ cups frozen seedless grapes
- ½ cup Breyers Light Natural Vanilla ice cream
- 50 Pepperidge Farm Goldfish

The following is a list of 100-calorie snacks recommended by Dr. Smith:

- ¼ cup low-fat granola
- ¼ cup black beans with 1 tablespoon salsa and 1 tablespoon nonfat Greek yogurt
- 1 nonfat mozzarella cheese stick with ½ medium-size apple
- 4 slices of rolled smoked turkey dipped in 2 teaspoons honey mustard
- 3 dried apricots stuffed with 1 tablespoon crumbled blue cheese

- 2 graham cracker squares topped with 1 teaspoon peanut butter and sprinkled with cinnamon
- 2 roasted plum tomatoes sliced and topped with 2 tablespoons bread crumbs and a sprinkle of parmesan
- 1 potato, baked
- ½ cup raisin bran
- ½ English muffin with 2 tablespoons low-fat cottage cheese and 3 slices cucumber
- 3 cups of air-popped popcorn
- 1 hard-boiled egg with salt and pepper
- 10 cashews
- 1½ cups sugar snap peas
- 8 small shrimp with 3 tablespoons cocktail sauce

CONCLUSION

Losing weight is a gradual process that requires careful attention to diet and exercise. Unfortunately, after an initial period of weight loss, the body often stops responding to new and healthier habits, called a plateau, and is unable to reach its ultimate goal. The SHRED program is specially designed to help frustrated dieters break through the weight-loss plateau.

With its six distinct weeks—Prime, Challenge, Transformation, Ascend, Cleanse, and Explode—SHRED incorporates a wide variety of food, beverages, and exercises that are essential to shredding unwanted fat. People who follow the SHRED plan, whom Dr. Smith calls SHREDDERS, gain confidence, mental strength, and valuable knowledge about diet, exercise, and health.

SHREDDERS learn the importance of meal spacing, staggering their meals and snacks throughout the day in order to eliminate periods of intense hunger and to maintain healthy levels of hormones in the blood stream. In addition, SHREDDERS learn the difference between snacking and indulging. They learn to vary their food choices, and discover how to use food and beverages to cleanse their livers. SHREDDERS also learn how to utilize exercise more effectively—by combining different types of activities and breaking workouts into multiple sessions.

Some people will finish SHRED after one cycle (six weeks), while others will move through several cycles of the program as they continue to work toward their weight-loss and health goals. For most, SHRED becomes a permanent lifestyle.

CPSIA information can be obtained at www.ICGtesting.com
Printed in the USA
LVOW13s1108161013

357194LV00001B/14/P